YOUR KNOWLEDGE HAS VALUE

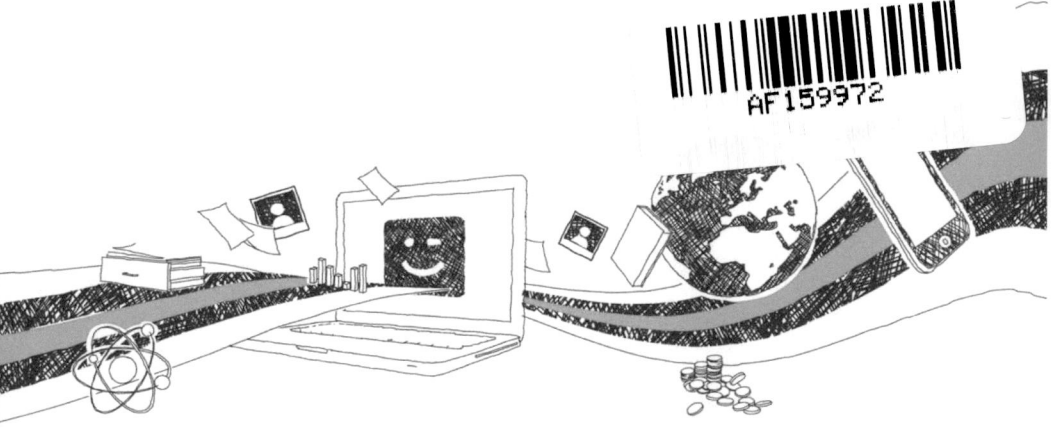

- We will publish your bachelor's and master's thesis, essays and papers

- Your own eBook and book - sold worldwide in all relevant shops

- Earn money with each sale

Upload your text at www.GRIN.com and publish for free

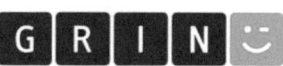

Bibliographic information published by the German National Library:

The German National Library lists this publication in the National Bibliography; detailed bibliographic data are available on the Internet at http://dnb.dnb.de .

This book is copyright material and must not be copied, reproduced, transferred, distributed, leased, licensed or publicly performed or used in any way except as specifically permitted in writing by the publishers, as allowed under the terms and conditions under which it was purchased or as strictly permitted by applicable copyright law. Any unauthorized distribution or use of this text may be a direct infringement of the author s and publisher s rights and those responsible may be liable in law accordingly.

Imprint:

Copyright © 2018 GRIN Verlag, Open Publishing GmbH
Print and binding: Books on Demand GmbH, Norderstedt Germany
ISBN: 9783668624665

This book at GRIN:

https://www.grin.com/document/388475

Patrick Kimuyu

Recent Medication for Peptic Ulcers

GRIN Publishing

GRIN - Your knowledge has value

Since its foundation in 1998, GRIN has specialized in publishing academic texts by students, college teachers and other academics as e-book and printed book. The website www.grin.com is an ideal platform for presenting term papers, final papers, scientific essays, dissertations and specialist books.

Visit us on the internet:

http://www.grin.com/

http://www.facebook.com/grincom

http://www.twitter.com/grin_com

Recent Medication for Peptic Ulcers

Name: Patrick Kimuyu

Introduction 2

Antibiotics 2
Clarithromycin 2
Indications 2
Side effects 2
Amoxicillin 3
Medications for Blocking Acid Production 4
Omeprazole 4
Indications 4
Side effects 4
Contraindications 4
Lansoprazole 5
Indications 5
Side effects 5
Contraindications 5
Cimetidine 5
Side effects 6
Contraindications 6

Conclusion 6

Bibliography 7

Introduction

Peptic ulcer has become one of the leading gastrointestinal (GIT) disorders. This phenomenon is attributable to the causes of the ulcers, especially Helicobacter pylori (H. pylori) infections which are difficult to treat[1]. They are also caused by acid production from the gastric lining. Therefore, treatment with recent medication depends on the cause of peptic ulcers. Currently, there are different forms of medication used for treating peptic ulcers comprising of antibiotics, acid blockers, antacids, and cytoprotective agents. This article provides a comprehensive discussion on recent medication for peptic ulcers.

Antibiotics

Antibiotics are used to eradicate H. pylori bacteria which cause sores in the GIT lining, especially the stomach and intestines. Currently, there are several regimens that have been approved for the treatment of peptic ulcer disease. One of these regimens is the triple therapies comprising of Clarithromycin and amoxicillin as the principal antibiotics[2].

Clarithromycin

Clarithromycin is long-acting antibiotic that is formulated as tablets and suspension for oral administration. It belongs to macrolide antibiotics and its mechanism of action involves the inhibition of bacteria growth by preventing the formation of cellwall components.

Indications

This agent is indicated for the treatment of H. pylori infection in combination with other drugs. It is also used to treat other bacterial infections primarily bronchitis, pneumonia and infections of the skin, sinuses, ears, and throat.

Side effects

Side effects associated with clarithromycin include nausea, diarrhea, stomach pain, vomiting, and change in taste. Other mild side effects are heartburn and headache. It is also

---

[1] Huang, Jia-Qing, Sridhar Subbaramiah and Hunt Richard. "Role of Helicobacter pylori infection and non-steroidal anti-inflammatory drugs in peptic-ulcer disease: a meta-analysis." *The Lancet* 359, no. 9300 (2000): 14.

[2] Arcangelo, Virginia and Peterson Andrew. *Pharmacotherapeutics for Advanced Practice: A Practical Approach, Volume 536* (Philadelphia: Lippincott Williams & Wilkins, 2006) 377

known to cause serious side effects such as rash, itching, hives, difficulty in swallowing or breathing, blistering skin, fever, extreme tiredness, and muscle weakness. Other serious side effects include loss of appetite, yellowing of the skin, irregular heartbeat, double vision, and unusual bleeding. In addition, it causes swelling of the limbs, eyes, throat, lips, and the face.

Contraindications

Clarithromycin is not recommended for patients with jaundice, ventricular arrhythmia or extended QT interval. It is also not recommended for pregnant or lactating mothers. This drug interacts with a wide range of drugs including astemizole, colchicines, cisapride, ergotamine, lovastatin, terfenadine, simvastatin, and pimozide. Other medications that interact with clarithromycin are anticoagulants: warfarin; certain benzodiazepines: midazolam and triazolam alprazolam; calcium channel blockers: diltiazem, verapamil and amlodipine; bromocriptine; cholesterol lowering drugs: pravastatin and atorvastatin; diabetes medication: repaglinide, nateglinide, pioglitazone, and rosiglitazone; rifampin; sildenafil; tolterodine; tadalafil; and theophylline.

Amoxicillin

Amoxicillin is an antibiotic that is available in different formulations: tablet, capsule, pediatric drops, suspension, and chewable tablet. It belongs to the class of penicillin-like antibiotics; thus it kills H. pylori bacteria through inhibiting cellwall formation. As such, it prevents bacterial growth leading to its eradication.

Indications

Amoxicillin is combined with other medications to eliminate H. pylori infection[3]. It is also indicated for certain bacterial infections such as gonorrhea, pneumonia, bronchitis, and other bacterial infections of the urinary tract, throat, nose, ear, and skin.

Side effects

Some of the mild side effects that are associated to amoxicillin are diarrhea, vomiting and upset stomach. It is also known to cause serious side effects such as seizure, hives, unusual bleeding, yellowing of the eyes or skin, and excessive tiredness. Moreover, pale skin and lack of energy are also considered as serious side effects that are caused by amoxicillin.

Contraindications

---

[3] Buch, George. *Pharmacology ReCap 2.0 for Bachelor of Dentistry Students* (Gujarat: Quick Review of Pharmacology, 2010) 378.

Amoxicillin is known to interact with chloramphenicol and probenecid. It is also worth noting that amoxicillin is not recommended for patients with kidney disease, asthma, allergies, and phenylketonuria.

Medications for Blocking Acid Production

Treatment and management of peptic ulcer comprises of regimens that block acid production; a condition which is stimulated by H. pylori bacteria. Recent medications include omeprazole, lansoprazole, ranitidine, cimetidine, and famotidine.

Omeprazole

This medication belongs to the class of proton pump inhibitors[4]. It blocks the action of acid-producing cells in the stomach, in order to block the release of acid into the stomach, and prevent ulcerations on the gastric linings.

Indications

Omeprazole is indicated for the treatment of ulcers caused by H. pylori bacteria. It also treats Zollinger-Ellison syndrome, a condition characterized by excessive acid production in the stomach. In addition, omeprazole can be prescribed for the treatment of gastroesophageal reflux disease.

Side effects

Omeprazole causes mild and adverse side effects. Mild side effects associated with the drug are constipation, nausea, headache, and vomiting. On the other hand, severe side effects include rash, itching, hives, dizziness, seizures, muscle spasms, diarrhea, and fever[5]. Other side effects are irregular heartbeat, excessive tiredness, difficulty in swallowing, hoarseness, and swelling of the ankles, eyes and throat.

Contraindications

Omeprazole interacts with a wide range of medications including ampicillin, warfarin, diazepam, atazanavir, clopidogrel, cilostazol, and digoxin. It also interacts with diuretics, saquinavir, Methotrexate, taclolimus, phenytoin, and cyclosporine. Moreover, antifungal medications are known to interact with omeprazole.

---

[4] Williams, Beverly and Paul Pauline. *Brunner & Suddarth's Textbook of Canadian Medical-surgical Nursing* (Philadelphia: Lippincott Williams & Wilkins, 2009), 1138.

[5] Watkins, Cynthia. *Pharmacology Clear & Simple: A Guide to Drug Classifications and Dosage Calculations.* (Philadelphia: F.A. Davis, 2013) 353.

Lansoprazole

Lansoprazole is a proton pump inhibitor that blocks acid production in the stomach during H. pylori infection[6]. It acts by blocking the mechanism involved in acid production by acid producing cells in the stomach; thus reducing the level of acid in the stomach and intestines.

Indications

Lansoprazole is used with other drugs for the treatment of ulcers caused by H. pylori. It is also used to treat heartburn and other conditions such as gastroesophageal reflux disease and Zollinger-Ellison syndrome.

Side effects

Side effects caused by lansoprazole are more or less the same as those caused by other proton pump inhibitors. These side effects include rash, headache, nausea, blistering of the skin, hoarseness, constipation, and fever[7]. Other side effects are seizures, severe diarrhea, dizziness, muscle spasms, and excessive tiredness. In some situations, this medication causes irregular heartbeat and swelling of the throat, face, eyes and the lips.

Contraindications

Lansoprazole interacts with ampicillin, ketoconazole, blood thinners, diuretics, theophylline and sucralfate. It is also known to interact with other medications such as digoxin, iron supplements, tacrolimus, and Methotrexate.

Cimetidine

Cimetidine is an over-the-counter medication which belongs to the class of H2 blockers[8]. This drug reduces the release of acid in the stomach by blocking the action of histamine which stimulates acid producing cells in the stomach lining. As a result, it relieves patients with peptic ulcers from pain and promotes healing.

Indications

---

[6] Williams, Beverly and Paul Pauline, 1138.

[7] Watkins, Cynthia. *Pharmacology Clear & Simple: A Guide to Drug Classifications and Dosage Calculations*. (Philadelphia: F.A. Davis, 2013) 353.

[8] Williams, Beverly and Paul Pauline. *Brunner & Suddarth's Textbook of Canadian Medical-surgical Nursing* (Philadelphia: Lippincott Williams & Wilkins, 2009), 1138.

Cimetidine is used to manage the symptoms associated with acid indigestion which is characterized by heartburn. In addition, this medication treats sour stomach, a condition associated with peptic ulcer disease.

Side effects

Cimetidine causes an array of side effects ranging from mild to severe conditions. In most cases, it causes drowsiness, headache, diarrhea, confusion, depression, nervousness, and excitement. It also causes hallucinations and dizziness, as well as breast enlargement in women[9].

Contraindications

In practice, cimetidine has been found to interact with metronidazole, diazepam, amoxipine, ptopranolol, lidocaine, amitriptyline, and ketoconazole. Other drugs that interact with cimetidine are warfarin, desipramine, theophylline, and nifedipine.

Conclusion

In a brief conclusion, recent medication for peptic ulcer disease comprises of a combination of drugs which address different conditions associated with the disease. Antibiotics eradicate H. pylori bacteria; whereas proton pump inhibitors and histamine blockers prevent acid production in the stomach to promote healing of the ulcers. On the other hand, antacids neutralize the acid in the stomach.

Bibliography

Arcangelo, Virginia and Peterson Andrew. *Pharmacotherapeutics for Advanced Practice: A Practical Approach, Volume 536*. Philadelphia: Lippincott Williams & Wilkins, 2006.

Buch, George. *Pharmacology ReCap 2.0 for Bachelor of Dentistry Students*. Gujarat: Quick Review of Pharmacology, 2010.

Huang, Jia-Qing, Sridhar Subbaramiah and Hunt Richard. "Role of Helicobacter pylori infection and non-steroidal anti-inflammatory drugs in peptic-ulcer disease: a meta-analysis." *The Lancet* 359, no. 9300 (2000): 14-24.

Watkins, Cynthia. *Pharmacology Clear & Simple: A Guide to Drug Classifications and Dosage Calculations*. Philadelphia: F.A. Davis, 2013.

Williams, Beverly and Paul Pauline. *Brunner & Suddarth's Textbook of Canadian Medical-surgical Nursing*. Philadelphia: Lippincott Williams & Wilkins, 2009.

YOUR KNOWLEDGE HAS VALUE

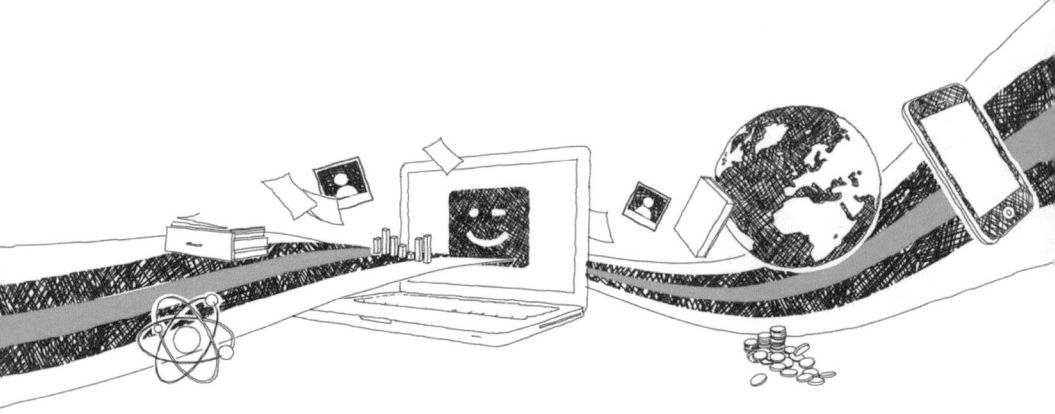

- We will publish your bachelor's and master's thesis, essays and papers

- Your own eBook and book - sold worldwide in all relevant shops

- Earn money with each sale

Upload your text at www.GRIN.com
and publish for free

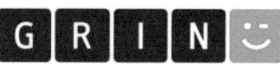